Thoughts Impact Your Health

Aries Ford Pemkiewicz
BS, RDN, LDN

Dedication

This book is dedicated to God for using me as a vessel to bring forth fruit. God is worthy of all glory and honor. My Prayer is that He calls me a Friend because I will do His Will.

John 15:14:16 (NKJ)

14 Ye are my friends, if ye do whatsoever I command you.

15 Henceforth I call you not servants; for the servant knoweth not what his lord doeth: but I have called you friends; for all things that I have heard of my Father I have made known unto you.

16 Ye have not chosen me, but I have chosen you, and ordained you, that ye should go and bring forth fruit, and *that* your fruit should remain: that whatsoever ye shall ask of the Father in my name, he may give it you.

*A*cknowledgements

To my spiritual leaders, my family and friends for all your loving support. I love you all very dearly and pray abundant blessings over your lives. A special thanks to my boot camp instructor.

Contents

$\mathcal{I}$ntroduction

You need this powerful book if you are seeking
better health. You must read this book if you are
suffering from a chronic disease or if you are at risk
for developing diabetes; high blood pressure or
heart disease which also includes having a family
history. Nothing matters when you are in poor
health. Your quality of life matters to me.
This book will provide you with the keys and
strategies to improve your health through thoughts,
speech and nutritional actions. Learn how to think
and speak your health into shape. I am your
Registered Dietitian Nutritionist. Say yes to a
healthier, stronger, energized body.

Key components include sample disease fighting
meal plans, how to reduce fat around your
abdomen, instructions for grocery shopping/ label
reading, portion sizes, proper nutrition as we age
and the real deal on how and why fasting can
impact your health at the cellular level.

Chapter 1

Thoughts Impact Your Health

*Y*our health is influenced by your thoughts and speech. Therefore, you have the power to speak life into your health. For example, our thoughts control the atmosphere around us and within us. What we speak also controls the atmosphere. You have the ability to change the way you think about your health, which will in turn transform your life. However, you need to learn how to rethink nutrition in order to transform your health. This book reveals powerful tools to jump start a healthier, stronger, energized body.

Purifying your thoughts and meditating on how consuming foods in their natural state will influence your health by allowing your body to heal at the cellular level. You will become healthier once you choose to eat healthier. Your new taste buds will follow once you tell your mind and body how good it will feel when you decide to take control of your health. You will experience increased energy, loss of stubborn fat cells and much better cholesterol, blood pressure and blood glucose control. We must eat to live and not live to eat. Excessive intake of high fat and sugary foods is not worth your life. Make the choice to think, speak and live healthy.

Many people suffer from diabetes, hypertension, cancer, obesity and over 25 million people have diabetes. Over 7 million people don't know they have it and over 79 million people have pre-diabetes (which is the medical term given to those who are on the verge of developing diabetes.) 68 million adults have high blood pressure and are taking blood pressure lowering drugs. 71 million people have bad cholesterol levels and more than 35% of the people in the United States are obese. Health risks are determined by using your weight and height to calculate a number called the body mass index (BMI). BMI under 18.5 = (underweight) and 18.5 - 24.9 = (healthy weight) and 25 - 29.9 = (overweight) and 30 or higher = (obese).

You can also use the waist to hip ratio to determine your risk especially for men with an abundance of muscle that are very active in sports. The BMI chart does not take into account muscle mass. Waist circumference is a good indicator of abdominal fat which is a predictor of risk for obesity related diseases. Overweight and obesity is caused by eating too many calories and inactivity. Health consequences include diabetes, coronary heart disease, cancer, high blood pressure, high lipid levels, stroke, liver and gallbladder disease, sleep apnea, osteoarthritis and gynecological problems. The initial treatment should be dietary changes. In other words, changing what we put in our mouths.

Health can be defined as the state of complete physical, mental and social well-being or the condition of being sound in body, mind and spirit. Healthy doesn't mean you have to weigh 100 lbs! Healthy can be losing 20 lbs if you are overweight (BMI > 25) or gaining 20 lbs if you are under weight (BMI < 18). I have counseled people and have seen the affects of losing even 10% or gaining 10%. I've seen huge improvements in lab values (blood work) and some people were able to lower their dose of medications or gained the ability to stop their meds with doctor's approval. What kinds of changes do we need to make? This change requires changes in our thought habits.
Say no to diabetes, heart disease, high blood pressure, high cholesterol, obesity, stroke risk and arthritis. What you speak matters. Your body says no to bad health every time you embrace good meaningful nutritional changes and put them into practice. The same goes for every time you think of eating a piece of fruit instead of a candy bar and modeling it. Your thoughts will and can change your behaviors. Your behaviors will in turn change your health.

Chapter 2

Nutrition Transformation

*J*ransform your nutrition *J*ransform your body

*J*ransform your health

Studies show that stress and consuming excessive, fat, sugar, sodium, genetically modified and processed foods contributes to inflammation which leads to chronic diseases. Therefore, we can win back our health by changing the way we think about stress related events and how we think about the foods we consume.

We can reduce our stress levels by listening to music, engaging in fun activities and simply giving our burdens to God. Stress if reduced when we realize and allow God to handle whatever is out of our control and praying for wisdom.

 Are you ready to change the way you think about the foods you eat. It is healthier to eat foods in their purest natural state without additives. Our bodies will obtain the most nutrients and disease fighting properties called antioxidants. Your daily intake should include 5-9 servings of colorful raw vegetables and fruits. Limit the amounts of bananas. Protein sources should include baked or grilled lean meats, beans and nuts. Choose rice and potatoes before bread and pasta. Bread, pasta and high calorie desserts should only be consumed once a week. Don't forget the water. Adequate hydration will also allow your cells to function at an optimum performance level to aid in your overall health.
No one likes to be hungry. I recommend combining non-starchy vegetables or fruits with a protein source during snack and meal times. It's best to eat vegetables a few hours before or after fruit. Fruits and vegetables consumed together will increase fermentation and intestinal gasses.

Eating protein helps to stabilize blood sugar levels, strengthen muscles and keep you feeling full longer. Reducing the amounts of bread and pasta will lower your risk for inflammation, diabetes, obesity and intestinal diseases.

Ezekiel 47:12(amp)
And on the banks of the river on both its sides, there shall grow all kinds of trees for food; their leaf shall not fade nor shall their fruit fail [to meet the demand]. Each tree shall bring forth new fruit every month, [these supernatural qualities being] because their waters came from out of the sanctuary. And their fruit shall be for food and their leaves for healing.

There are an abundance of healing properties in vegetables, fruits, tea leaves and water. Consuming foods in their natural state will improve your overall health dramatically.

Sample Menu (made a difference in my life)

6:30am Wake up to hydrate. Consume 16 oz of water upon getting up

8:00am –enjoy a cup of green or black tea with a dash of cinnamon

10am- 8 oz of water, 6 raw sweet peppers, 5 raw broccoli florets, ½ cup of baby carrots with 1 tbsp of blue cheese dressing and 15 almonds

12 noon-Grilled chicken on a bed of salad with 1 small baked potato. Add another serving of raw vegetables of choice. 16 oz of water

2:30pm-1 sliced apple with 2 tbsp of peanut butter or 1/2c of peanuts and 1 cup of green tea with a dash of cinnamon

5:00 pm- 3 oz Grilled salmon, 1/2 cup of rice pilaf, steamed green beans and
 ½ cup of sorbet. 8-16 oz water

7:00 pm- 15 almonds, 1 cup of grapes and 8 oz of water or decaf green tea

You can always substitute vegetarian protein sources for meats. Total water intake should at least be eight -8oz cups per day. This does not include tea.

This menu is not indicated for individuals who have diabetes. I recommend that you consult a Registered Dietitian for an individualized meal plan. Other benefits from this meal plan include a visible reduction in fat around your abdomen, release of impurities and healthier skin.

Chapter 3

Keys for Realigning Your Health

$\mathcal{T}$his chapter will help you to overcome your nutritional

challenges. Knowledge will align your sensory processing factors which will realign your health. I will provide you with the keys on how to transform your fitness levels, shop healthier, reduce processed food intake and determine portion sizes.

Grocery Shopping Keys
- Make a list to save time and money. It only makes sense to look at the sales paper to determine what's on sale first. Look in your cabinets and see what you really need from the sale items to start making healthy meals at home. Now you are ready to create a list to provide meals for the next 7 days or so. Consider vegetarian meals during the week as well.

- Start in the produce aisle first. Look for colorful, nutrient rich fruits and vegetables. Bright colors indicate more antioxidants which help to protect the body. Produce is also rich in fiber and very low in calories. Half of your lunch and dinner plate should be filled with selections from the produce aisle.

- Next we can look for dry items and save the cold items for last. We need to keep those items cold as long as possible.

- Shop for whole grain items such as breads, pasta, and rice. Don't forget the nuts and beans.

Now we can shop for lean skinless meats, fish and low fat and fat free dairy. You can also replace your dairy with rice or almond milk and green leafy vegetables. Lean meats include skinless chicken and turkey breast, beef cuts without marbling (fat), (sparingly) round steak tenderloin, sirloin tips and center cuts. Don't forget to keep raw meats on the bottom of the cart to prevent cross contamination.

Frozen items should be last in order to keep them frozen as long as possible during travel. You can shop for frozen unbreaded meats/fish, fruits, vegetables, whole grain breakfast items and sorbets. Sometimes frozen foods can be more cost effective, and they are packed with nutrients.

Try not to shop for foods that have a lot of added ingredients such as fat, sugar and salt such as : processed foods, boxed rice, pasta and potato mixes, canned soups, TV dinners, breaded meats and vegetables, bacon, sausage, tuna canned in oil, beans cooked in lard, vegetables cooked in cream or cheese sauces, fried vegetables, sweet rolls, doughnuts, pastries, biscuits, fried tortillas, sugar coated cereals, juices or drinks sweetened with sugar, fruit canned in heavy syrup, 2% or whole milk, regular cheese, yogurt with sugar, hot dogs, and meat with skin.

These foods are high in calories, fat, sodium and or sugar. Moderation is the key as well as finding these choices with reduced sodium, sugar and fat.
Canned foods tend to be high in sodium. Try to purchase reduced sodium or no added salt. You can also rinse your vegetables thoroughly to remove the sodium before consuming. Purchase snacks that are low in fat, sodium, sugar and free of trans fats or hydrogenated oils. Good snacks include bite size raw fruits and vegetables, unsalted pretzels, animal crackers, Jello or pudding. Sherbet and sorbet are good choices. Good snack choices include items that contain less than 5 grams of fat per serving.

Look for these basic label readings at a glance while shopping. Fat and sodium content is the most important items to read on the food label during shopping if you are new at reading labels and want to save time. You can worry about the serving size and carbohydrate count when you get home. Items high in fat will most likely be high in calories. Eating too much fat makes us fat. Healthy eating means reducing the fat and sodium we consume. You also want to be familiar with high fiber choices. Choose food items with greater than 5 grams of fiber per serving.

Don't forget that it is also important to know what's in your food. Let me show you what to look for on a label. Find a label in your kitchen and follow along with me.

Serving size- determines the amount of calories and nutrients in one serving. You have to add more calories if you decide to eat more or the entire package. The same idea goes for fat, sodium and carbohydrates as well.

Fat grams- Compare products and choose foods with the least amount of total fat grams- less than 5 grams of fat per serving for snack foods.

Sodium- Try to choose foods lowest in sodium. 140mg is a good goal per serving.

Carbohydrates- One serving of carbohydrates is equivalent to 15 grams of carbohydrates. A sugar gram is just a component of carbohydrates. Carbohydrates break down into sugar. Seek a dietitian if you want a personalized carbohydrate controlled meal plan.

Fiber- Try to choose items with 5 grams or more per serving.

<u>Keys to overcome unhealthy partnerships and nutritional challenges</u>

These suggestions will help to control blood pressure, cholesterol and blood glucose levels.

1- Don't drink your calories! Drink water or unsweetened drinks only. Our bodies need at least 6 to 8 glasses of water a day. Water also helps to jump start your metabolism and is required and helps many functions at the cellular level. Sweetened drinks have a quick impact on your blood sugar levels and provide you with lots of empty calories that can cause you to gain weight. I've seen people lose 1 to 2 pounds a week just by stopping regular sodas.

2- Don't skip meals! What do we do when we skip a meal? We inhale the entire kitchen table the next time we sit down to eat. This causes us to take in extra calories that will cause weight gain. Instead, try to have a small healthy snack if you are unable to eat within a reasonable time frame.

3- Think balance. Eat a variety of foods at meal time. Don't eat an entire plate of mac-n-cheese for dinner. Be sure to include meat or vegetable protein, starch, vegetables and fruit for dessert. You body requires a variety of foods to provide vital nutrients to jump start metabolism and initiate other functions at the cellular level.

4- Watch those portions! The plate method is the easiest way to watch portions. No, you cannot pile the plate up like a mountain peak. Half of your plate should be non-starchy vegetables other than beans, corn and potatoes (these are considered starches.) A serving of starch is usually 1/3 to ½ cup serving. You should include 3 oz of meat (which is the size of the palm of your hand) or vegetable protein. Vegetarians are allowed more vegetable proteins or protein substitutes to meet their protein needs. They include beans, nuts, soy, tofu, hummus, peanut butter, almond butter and cheese. A ½ ounce of nuts, 1 tablespoon of peanut butter, ¼ cup of beans or 1 egg is equal to 1 ounce of meat protein. Most people need at least 6 ounces of protein per day. These are general serving guidelines. Please consult a registered dietitian for a personal meal plan and the right serving sizes to meet your individual needs.

5- Balance your carbohydrates (starches such as pasta, rice, bread, beans, potatoes, and corn), fruit, milk and sweets. It's very important that we don't over indulge on these foods. Please contact a registered dietitian or myself if you have diabetes for an individualized meal plan.

6- Watch portions of meat and choose lean meats. 3 oz is a general guideline or the size of the palm of your hand. Choose baked, broiled or grilled meats instead of fried. Watch the cheese. Try adding more vegetable proteins to your meals like peanut butter, nuts and beans instead of meat a few times per week.

7- Eat less fat. Choose lower fat items at restaurants and at the grocery store. Watch servings of salad dressings, butter/margarine, sour cream, cream cheese, cheese, whole milk, and gravies, processed meats (sausage, bacon, and hotdogs.) Choose foods that are baked or grilled. Try rice or almond milk instead of whole milk.

8- Watch the salt. Try not to add salt at the table and reduce processed foods, meats, TV dinners, instant flavored potato/rice boxed mixes and soups. Choose fresh or frozen vegetables most of the time or rinse off the canned vegetables at home.

9- Read food labels and choose lower fat and sodium choices. Use this same guideline while eating out. Take half of your meal home with you or share with your lunch or dinner partner.

10- Try to use other seasonings while cooking instead of salt and butter. Garlic powder, lemon pepper, onion powder and lemon juice are some good substitutions that add flavor. You can also season foods with a variety of vegetables such as colorful peppers and onions.

Keys for a healthy weight loss for individuals with a BMI over 27
- Eat at least 3 times a day.
- Try not to go more than 5 hrs between meals
- Know when you are hungry. A good rule is a stomach growl.
- Drink a glass of water before each meal and drink water during your meals.
- Don't eat in front of the TV. Your stomach sends the signal to the brain that you are full, but your brain is occupied watching TV which increases your chances of over eating.
- Use smaller plates and bowls.
- Eat slowly and put your fork or spoon down while you chew. Cut your food one bite at a time.
- Brush your teeth after you eat.
- Cook when you are not hungry and drink water while you cook.
- Be careful of emotional eating- Don't eat because you are bored or sad. Read an inspirational book (the bible), call a friend, listen to music or take a walk.

Nutritional Keys For Successful Aging
It is important to maintain your health at all ages. There are many concerns for older adults as we age. Your metabolism will begin to slow down and your taste may be altered. Older Americans experience a reduction in the ability to absorb key nutrients, dehydration and a sluggish digestive system. Therefore, it is imperative to consume adequate water, B vitamins, fiber and less fat. It is important to eat less calories if you are overweight and nutrient dense or high calorie foods if you are underweight. Simple walking exercises are suggested to strength then your heart and bones.

<u>15 minute activity keys to transform your body</u>

Engaging in 15 minutes of daily activity can transform the way your body looks and feels. You can achieve this without equipment. I would like to introduce three basic exercises that will make a huge difference in your energy, lab values, fat loss and muscle gain. Perform these basic exercises in 30-60 second intervals. Thirty seconds of exercise and sixty seconds of rest, for a total of 15 minutes.

1. Jumping Jacks- provides an overall workout
2. Alternate high and low plank- provides arms and abdominal toning
3. Swats – provides thigh and buttock toning
4. Leg lifts- lay on your back and lift your legs 6 inches and hold

Don't forget to check with your doctor before starting a new exercise regimen. Remember to start slow and always stop when you feel abnormally tired.

This simple 15 minute plan can jump start your weight loss, maintain your weight and prevent further weight gain. Other benefits include:
- Preventing and managing health conditions and disease, strengthen bones to reduce falls, improves heart health, and improves blood sugar and blood pressure levels as well.
- Boost energy levels by delivering more oxygen to your tissues.
- Improves your mood, releases stress and improves confidence. You look better and feel better about yourself.
- Promotes better sleep at night.

Exercising large muscle groups is an effective way to burn fat and gain muscle. Add weight baring exercises to your weekly workouts. One pound weight loss per week is equivalent to burning 3500 calories. That's 500 calories a day or reducing you food intake by 500 calories per day.

Food and Activity Log
(keep a journal of everything you eat and drink. Logging your exercise is equally important. Start today) Use this space

Chapter 4

Abundant Healing

$\mathcal{M}$ost people do not understand the impact of fasting on your health. This chapter will give you a closer look at the power behind fasting and increase your knowledge to impact your overall physical health. You can actually remove risk factors for disease

Studies show that a reduction in IGF1 can dramatically reduce your risk factors for cancer and diabetes. IGFI (Insulin growth factor 1) is reduced when we fast. Our bodies were created to fast. There are many benefits to fasting, such as purging diseases, increased brain cell development, optimal fat reduction abundant healing, and age reduction. It is suggested to fast every three months to maintain low levels of IGF1.

There are the three major contributors to developing disease. We feed disease or increase our risk when we consume a diet high in calories, fat, sugar and protein. These groups of foods increase the growth of Insulin Growth Factor 1 hormone(IGF1).

This is how it works. You body reduces IGF1 after you have fasted 3-4 days. This also reduces the growth of disease causing cells and these particular cells begin to repair themselves. Your brain will begin to increase the number of brain cells and neuron growth and the liver begins to burn a greater amount of fat. Therefore, it is very beneficial to reduce calories, sugar, fat and high intake of meats. We should consume a diet low in sugar, fat, sodium and chose vegetable protein sources with most of our meals.

Abundant Healing takes place during a fast. Every cell in your body prepares to give God glory when you decide to fast. Jesus allows your cells to shift into a spiritual mode to sustain your body. Our cells and organs will run different cycles to provide fuel for physical maintenance. We obtain fuel from carbohydrates, fats and protein. However, our bodies were made to shift into modes to provide all of these. Your liver was designed to undergo gluconeogenesis and lipogenesis. This is a metabolic pathway that releases fat and glucose into the blood stream to be used for energy. God created gluconeogenesis and lipogenesis for us. Genesis 1:31 "And God saw everything that he had made, and, behold, it was very good. And the evening and the morning were the sixth day". Genesis 2:2"

God rested on the 7th day. Fasting also gives our bodies rest from all the daily toxins we take in from not consuming food in its natural state. We can't control the chemicals place in our foods but we can control the types of foods we purchase and consume. We need to be selective in our food choices, cooking methods and portion sizes. You make these decisions on a daily basis.

Benefits of Fasting

Better health, promotes healing, used to honor God and to increase spiritual breakthroughs. Fasting can also increase your relationship with Jesus and the anointing on your life to do the will of God (Isaiah 61). Sometimes a fast can expedite the answers to questions or request that you have asked God.

The length of your fast should be lead by the Holy Spirit. However "The Daniel Fast" is the most common fast. It is a 21 day fast with a focus on fruits and vegetables. I recommend you purchase my other book called "Vessels of Gold and Silver" and "Godly Feast" for more detailed information regarding time frames, examples of different types of non-food fast and verses related to spiritual fasting. I recommend that you start with a 3-4 day fast if this is your first time. This time frame will at least allow for the reduction of IGF1 which will facilitate a physical and spiritual purge.

Some people time frames vary from 1 day to 40 days. The time frame is up to you and the Holy Spirit. However, starting with 3-4 days will be most effective for physical results including a reduction in abdominal fat, rejuvenating your skin and overall energy. Please take caution if you are pregnant, underweight or have a medical condition that does not permit you to fast. Consult your physician and seek a dietitian or me for an idividualized consultation.

Listed below are protein substitutes.

You can replace meats with these foods:
1/2 ounce of nuts or 23 almonds

1 tablespoon of peanut butter or other nut butters

1/2 cup of beans

1/2 cup brown rice

High protein cereal (grams of protein and serving size will

vary. Read the food label)

Take a moment to plan a meal with these protein sources

-

-

-

-

-

Keys For a Fasting Breakthrough

- Spend more time in prayer, worship/praise, reading the bible and memorizing scriptures during the fasting time frame or in place of omitted meal times. Remain in God's presence

- Don't be afraid to ask according to God's will. Ask for the things that God would want you to have for His glory. 1 john 5:14

- Ask in confidence. In Jesus Name. 1 john 5:14

- Keep asking until the answer comes. Mat 7:7-8

- Don't give up. 1 Thess 5:17 Pray without ceasing

- Pray for wisdom. Proverbs 4:7

- Have faith in God. Mark 11:22

- Touch and agree with someone. Mat 18:19

  Again I say unto you, That if two of you shall agree on earth as touching any thing that they shall ask, it shall be done for them of my Father which is in heaven.

- Ask for forgiveness. Psalms 51

- Remain in obedience and don't break God's laws. Psalms 119:4

- Read scriptures that support your desires from God and memorize them.

- Psalms 1:2 But his delight *is* in the law of the LORD; and in his law doth he meditate day and night.

Miracles, signs and wonders come by fasting. Jesus fasted to honor God, thank God, Glorify God and expedite what was needed for those seeking healing. Healing is required by the mind, body and spirit. Fasting provides miracle breakthroughs are well as disease fighting cellular mechanisms to powerfully explode throughout your body. Fasting can heal your body physically at the cellular level. Other benefits include increasing your spiritual time with God, increasing good nutritional habits along with discipline and self control. We are to present ourselves as a living sacrifice and we are the temple of God. Your life and health depends on Jesus. Fasting allows us to abide in Him. He's able to purge the bad fruit and bring forth more good fruit. Jesus is the true vine.

John 15:1-7(KJV)
I am the true vine, and my Father is the husbandman.

[2] Every branch in me that beareth not fruit he taketh away: and every *branch* that beareth fruit, he purgeth it, that it may bring forth more fruit.

[3] Now ye are clean through the word which I have spoken unto you.

[4] Abide in me, and I in you. As the branch cannot bear fruit of itself, except it abide in the vine; no more can ye, except ye abide in me.

[5] I am the vine, ye *are* the branches: He that abideth in me, and I in him, the same bringeth forth much fruit: for without me ye can do nothing.

[6] If a man abide not in me, he is cast forth as a branch, and is withered; and men gather them, and cast *them* into the fire, and they are burned.

[7] If ye abide in me, and my words abide in you, ye shall ask what ye will, and it shall be done unto you.

Our health is indeed within our speech. You can ask Him to restore your health, if you abide in Him. Speak good health out loud during your fast and watch God!

DISCLAIMER

This book is written to promote nutrition, health and healing. Please seek a professional dietitian before starting a nutrition plan.

ABOUT THE AUTHOR

Please visit my website at
www.AriesFord.org
For nutrition consults and many other
inspirational reading materials.

You may have seen appearances
by Aries on WXII 12
"Parents balancing work and family",
"Moms saving Time",
TCP and Triad Fitness and Health Magazines.